AND BABY MAKES FOUR

A Trimester-by-Trimester Guide to a Baby-Friendly Dog

Penny Scott-Fox, CPDT

Illustrated by Ingrid Kallick

And Baby Makes Four

Project Team
Editor: Stephanie Fornino
Copy Editor: Joann Woy
Illustrator: Ingrid Kallick
Designer: Stephanie Krautheim

T.F.H. Publications
President/CEO: Glen S. Axelrod
Executive Vice President: Mark E. Johnson
Publisher: Christopher T. Reggio
Production Manager: Kathy Bontz

T.F.H. Publications, Inc.
One TFH Plaza
Third and Union Avenues
Neptune City, NJ 07753

Printed and bound in China

07 08 09 10 11   1 3 5 7 9 8 6 4 2

Library of Congress Cataloging-in-Publication Data

Scott-Fox, Penny.
   And baby makes four : A trimester-by-trimester guide to a baby-friendly dog / Penny Scott-Fox.
      p. cm.
   ISBN 0-7938-0567-8 (alk. paper)
   1. Dogs—Training. 2. Dogs—Behavior. 3. Dogs—Social aspects. 4. Children and animals. I. Title.
   SF431.S39 2007
   636.7'089689142—dc22
                                              2006022431

This book has been published with the intent to provide accurate and authoritative information in regard to the subject matter within. While every precaution has been taken in preparation of this book, the author and publisher expressly disclaim responsibility for any errors, omissions, or adverse effects arising from the use or application of the information contained herein. The techniques and suggestions are used at the reader's discretion and are not to be considered a substitute for veterinary care. If you suspect a medical problem consult your veterinarian.

The Leader In Responsible Animal Care For Over 50 Years!™

www.tfh.com

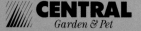

Table of
Contents

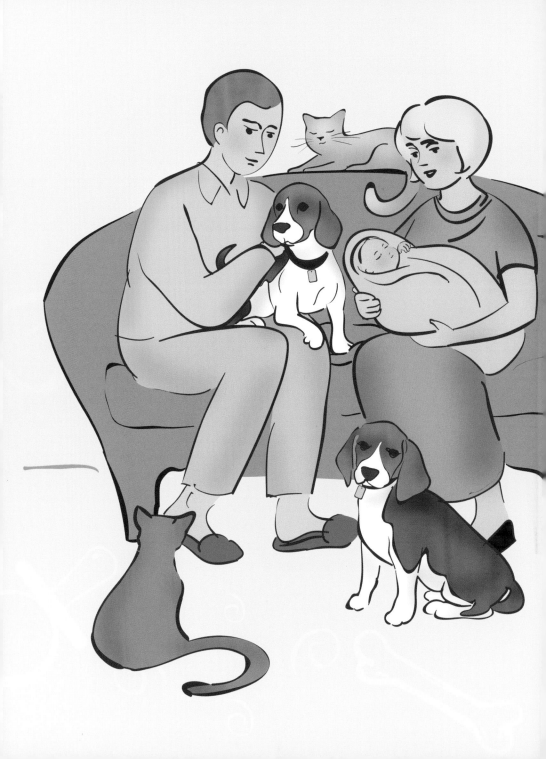

INTRODUCTION

It is said that necessity is the mother of invention. Considering the inspiration for this book, the phrase is more than apt.

I became pregnant with my son, Scott, in the summer of 1998. One of the first things that occurred to me when my doctor shared the happy news, aside from whether our baby would be healthy, was what our "four-legged kids" would think. My husband and I are the extremely proud parents of two delightful cats, Chenega and Kenaitze, plus Poppy and Caliban, our charming, irrepressible Beagles.

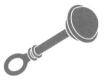

I had serious reservations about how each of these very individual, quirky characters would relate to our soon-to-arrive son, and I knew that I would have to address them, but as it turned out, I couldn't give any of that much thought initially. I had other, much more serious concerns. My first trimester was a nightmare, the details of which you will be spared.

It was during my second trimester that my thoughts turned to our animals and when the idea for this book came to me. I worked at the Pasadena Humane Society & Society for the Prevention of Cruelty to Animals (SPCA), where I was in my third year as an adoption counselor, matching pets with people and training to become the behavior specialist that I am now. During my time there, I had started to take note of something I hadn't observed before: the number of cats and dogs being turned into our shelter because the owner family was expecting. As I looked further into the subject, I began to realize that this is a problem of huge proportions and needless choices. Across the country, dogs, cats, and other pets are discarded in staggering numbers by families with unfounded fears about newborns and domestic animals living together.

Accurate statistics that describe this phenomenon are difficult to come by. Shelters are not always told the actual reason a pet is being given away. However, a reasonable conclusion didn't require much extrapolation. Presently, more than 5,000 animal shelters operate in the United States. My informal though informed research on the "pregnancy problem" in Pasadena clearly suggested that the pets destroyed or rehomed nationally each year would number in the tens of thousands. Just as alarming, in my research I learned that people can often be uncompromising on the subject. Misled by bad information—about, say, the so-called danger of Labradors jumping up or cats with toxoplasmosis—as far as they are concerned, it's out you go, Rover (and/or Fluffy).

I feel strongly that if we ask our pets to live with us, then it is only fair to prepare them for the great changes a baby brings to a household. Animals devote their lives to their owners, and they cannot suddenly be perceived as a threat. The arrival of a newborn is an intense time for everyone, and the very least we can do as responsible pet owners is to give our animals a chance.

Having a baby doesn't mean that you have to give your pet away. Put another way, in the words of a bumper sticker created by the National Canine Defence League in England, "Dogs are for life, not just for Christmas." I hope this book will be helpful to you and that you have much success in preparing your pet for the arrival of your baby. Again, I know it may be hard work, and it may be frustrating, but it will be so worth the effort. The program offered in this book is essential for your baby's safety, your peace of mind, and your pet's health and happiness. He will get to stay home with the people he loves, not be given up to a shelter and rehomed.

This book is going to focus mainly on dogs, but not because I don't love cats. Cats are just infinitely easier and don't need much work to adjust to a newborn. Don't worry, though—I have devoted the last chapter entirely to cats.

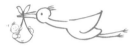

Did You Know?

Thousands of pets are given up to shelters annually because families assume that they won't be able to adjust to a new baby in the house.

HOW DO DOGS VIEW BABIES?

The majority of dogs do not view infants as a threat. However, they are susceptible to changes in their environment and routine. Change is not easy for a dog. It can alter his perception of his relationship with his human parents, leading to what he thinks is diminished affection and potentially causing more attention-seeking behavior. New parents may thus perceive his actions as aggression toward their baby.

The more you prepare your dog for the arrival of an infant, the better the bonding between baby and dog will be, and the more relaxed the new parents will be. Surely, having invited a dog to spend his life with you, it makes sense to prepare him for the changes that are about to happen. And make no mistake, a baby means serious changes to the environment and daily routine in any home.

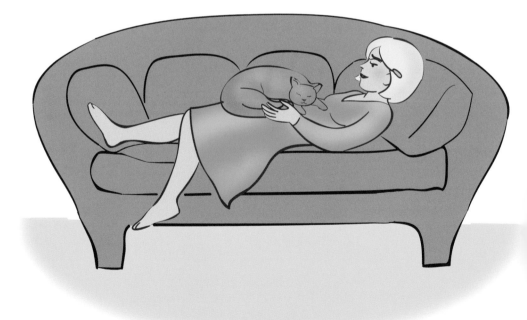

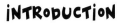

THE CHILD-PET BOND

Although this book focuses largely on dog behavior, I do have to share this story with you about our cats. While I was pregnant, Chenega and Kenaitze, both males, spent a lot of their time on my stomach, purring away. As my pregnancy progressed, Chenega became more and more cuddly. When Scott had the hiccups, I would grab one of the cats and put him on my tummy. The purring would stop the hiccups—which, as all expectant mothers know, is a decidedly uncomfortable in-womb sensation. After Scott was born, the cats already knew him and would sleep next to him at any opportunity, and when he got the hiccups, Chenega would jump up next to him. Naturally, the hiccups would stop immediately.

Perhaps not surprisingly, my son's first two words, both directed at Chenega, were "Mama" and "Neega." Needless to say, I am Mama now, but I wasn't for a couple of frustrating though amusing weeks! To this day, the bond between Scott and the two cats is extraordinary.

At this point, it should be noted that not all dogs (or cats) are born to live with babies. If, for example, your pet has exhibited any aggressiveness toward infants in the past or is skittish about even the smallest change, then he should be evaluated by a professional trainer before you undertake the program outlined in this book. Should that evaluation indicate that your dog is incapable of living with a baby, then I am truly sorry, and it is better that he be rehomed.

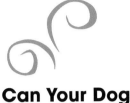

Can Your Dog Live With a Baby?

If you are unsure of whether your dog can live with a baby, contact a professional trainer for help.

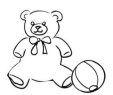

Poppy and Caliban, our Beagles, are among the great majority of animals who *can* be prepared for newborns, and I want to tell you something about them. As a breed, Beagles are not simple. They may be small and cute, but by instinct they are hunting dogs and would happily kill a rabbit or squirrel in a heartbeat. Both dogs are from a Beagle rescue, and both have issues of one sort or another. (Not all dogs from a shelter or rescue have been abused; some just run away, and the owners do not come looking for them for a number of reasons.)

Poppy was seven when Scott was born, extremely nervous and sound sensitive and totally overbonded to me. To this day, she can be aggressive when strangers approach, particularly men, as well as territorial in the house when people have the temerity to visit. She would bark at the sound of a pin dropping if she could. However, because of our relationship, she listened and was easy to train. Her training is ongoing, in fact. Such is life with a Beagle.

Caliban was four when Scott was born. He was and remains confident and easygoing, a friend to anyone as long as they feed him. He was hit by a car as a puppy, which shattered his rear left leg and hip. Fortunately, the accident never diminished his happy-go-lucky spirit. Caliban is also quite the clown, willing to steal anything in order to elicit a chase. He is obsessed with squeaky things and socks left untended

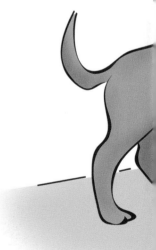
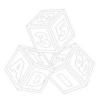

mere seconds out of the clothes dryer. Food overrides everything for Caliban, except when he is chasing cats.

Both dogs have been through a reward-based, group, basic obedience class. They both sit, down, stay, walk on a slack leash, and come when called. They are not super-trained dogs,

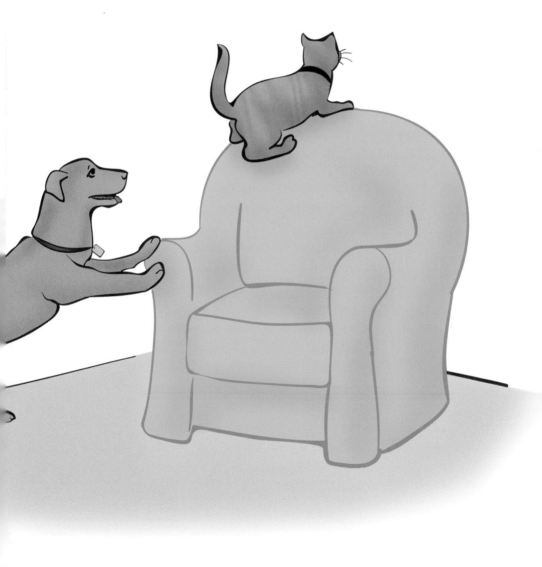

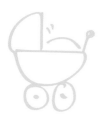

just great family pets who get along with Scott beautifully.

Using my family's experiences with our dogs and our home as a laboratory, I've created procedures to help keep devoted dogs at home where they belong and saved from an uncertain, potentially tragic fate.

HOW THIS BOOK IS ORGANIZED

The program and procedures in this book are organized to coincide with the trimesters of a pregnancy for a simple reason. Each trimester brings its own unique challenges. The first trimester, unless you are exceptionally lucky, is the worst, thanks to morning sickness and dramatic hormonal changes. It is the most anxiety-inducing time of your pregnancy. Thus, during the first trimester, the least amount of behavioral modification is required. The second trimester is typically the most pleasant and comfortable, and so you will have the most time and motivation to do the majority of the training. As you wind down in the final trimester, when feelings of excitement mix with apprehension, you are equipped with all the paraphernalia—stroller, car seat, baby lotions, high chair, nursery—that you will use to practice for baby. At the same time, you will be taking the behavior modification techniques you learned in the first and second trimesters and practicing with your dog for the arrival of baby.

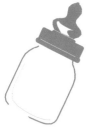

The procedures outlined in this book are as simple and straightforward as I can make them. You may find that they are a lot of work, and you may find them frustrating, but believe me, once your baby arrives, life will turn upside down. The time to start working on this is *before* the baby is born, not after, when it may be too late.

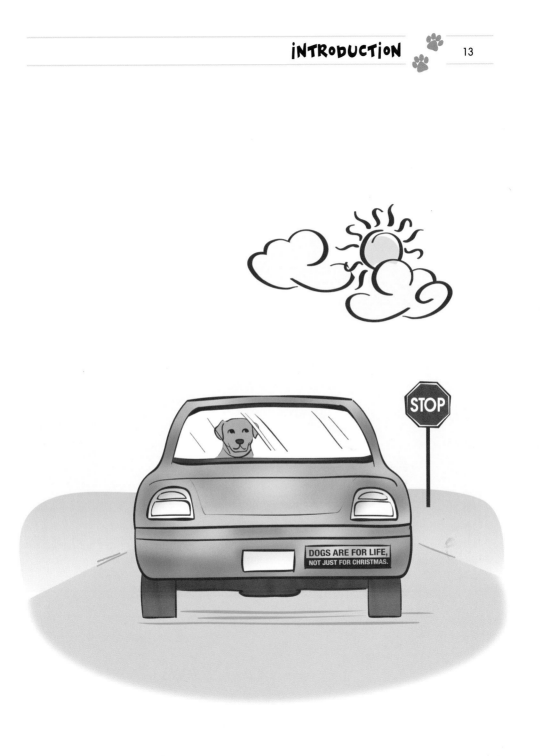

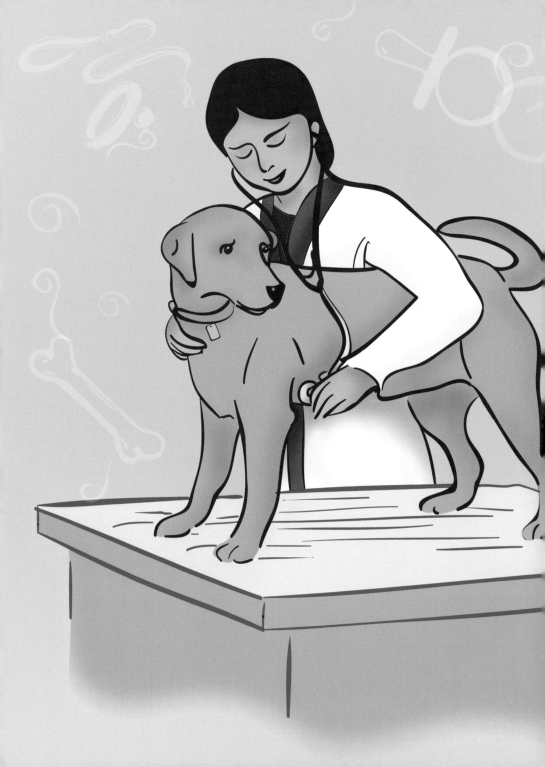

1

THE FIRST TRIMESTER:

Health Check and
Status Reduction Program

It is quite common for the pet in the house to be the "firstborn" who suddenly finds his world turned upside down when that little pink thing shows up. At this stage of your pregnancy, you now have nine months or less to change your dog's behavior, to keep his world spinning on its axis, and to graduate him from Number-One Spoiled Brat to the loving, happy, welcoming family pet whom you surely want.

TAKE YOUR DOG TO THE VET

During the first trimester, it is vital that you take your dog to your vet to have a full checkup, get up to date with shots, and make sure that he is in general good health. A few diseases can be passed from dogs to babies, among them roundworms, hookworms, and leptospirosis, so it is important to keep shots and wormings current. With all the doctor appointments you are going through, one more for your dog won't make much difference, and it could be a welcome break from all the stuff you have to do for the baby!

Take your dog to the vet for a full checkup and to make sure he's up to date with his shots.

IMPLEMENT STATUS REDUCTION PLAN

Newly expectant couples worry about how their "old baby" is going to get along with the real one, and so they should. Dogs are fantastic in many ways, but not even with the best training in the world can they be anything more than what they are.

Let's look at things from a dog's point of view. First, dogs are pack-oriented, social animals. Allowing them into our lives makes them part of *our* pack. In the wolf world, there is always a leader in the pack—the alpha. The alpha dog gets the best sleeping area, first pick at any available food, the right to go first through narrow spaces, and finally, respect and submission from the rest of the pack. Now, transpose your dog into your family life by answering these questions:

- Is he confused as to whether he is the leader?
- Does he sleep in/on your bed?

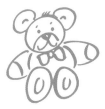

- Does he get fed before anyone else in the house?
- Does he pull while on leash?
- Does he respond to commands only when he feels like it?
- Is he possessive of food, toys, or trash?
- Are there any signs of aggression if you want to move him?
- Does he win all games?

If you answered yes to any of these questions, then you should begin the work of status reduction. Although both dominant and confident dogs can interact with an infant perfectly, it is important to set boundaries for your dog so that he understands what his role is in the household. Status reduction actually has nothing to do with dominance. It is about opening lines of communication between you and your dog in a way that he will understand—namely, teaching him that there is no free lunch. In other words, from here on out, your dog must earn everything he needs in life, rather than receive it for free. (One great way to teach your dog that he must earn his living is to have him sit or perform some other command before giving him his food or a treat.)

Although all dogs are opportunists, they prefer for you to be in charge. Being the leader is tough on a dog. At those times when you take control, he has to re-assert himself all over again. How exhausting! It is much easier for the dog to know where he stands right from the beginning, and his status should always be consistent. A newborn is not much of a threat to a dog—remember, change is what they don't like, not babies. (And by the way, more often than not, dogs bite parents, not babies.)

Begin the status reduction program described below as soon as possible during your pregnancy so that you feel confident that you have control over your dog. It is never too soon to start a status-reduction program. It's never too late, either!

Ignore Your Dog

Disregard any whining, pawing, staring, or other means to get your attention. Do not look at, speak to, or touch your dog. When he demands attention other than for a bathroom break outside, pretend he doesn't exist. Naturally, you must give your dog attention every day, but from now on it must be initiated by you.

Give Nothing Away for Free

Your dog should earn *everything* he wants. For example, he must obey a command such as *sit* before going outside, getting a treat, or eating dinner. Reserve at least half of his daily food allowance for rewards during training. Also, have extra-tasty treats (cheese is good) to give for especially nice behavior.

Serve Dinner on Schedule

Prepare your dog's dinner at the same time that you fix your own, and then eat yours while allowing him to observe. If necessary, leash him away from the table to prevent him from jumping up. Ignore any attempts to get your attention while you are eating, *and absolutely, positively do not feed him from the*

FIRST TRIMESTER CHECKLIST

1. Take dog to vet

2. Implement status reduction program

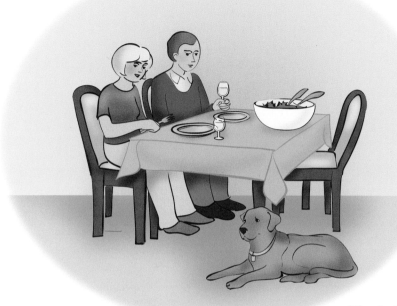

When implementing your status reduction plan, refrain from feeding your dog from the table.

table! When you are finished eating, you may add scraps from your plate to his bowl. Remember, only after you are finished eating should you feed him.

Establish Sleeping Quarters

Do not allow your dog to sleep in your bedroom. If your baby is in your room for nighttime feedings or perhaps sleeping there because of health concerns, such as colic, it will be easier all around if the dog is not present. No ifs, ands, or buts here, even if he already has established himself in your bedroom. He should have his own bed area, separate from all human members of the family.

If your dog is already used to sleeping in your bedroom, you must immediately take control of the situation. Set up his bed in another room, and close your bedroom door. Some dogs will bark or whine, but stand firm and ignore this behavior. It will pass. The longest I have known a dog to continue barking or whining when shut out of his owners' bedroom is four days.

Teach Basic Commands

Train your dog to obey basic commands such as *come, down, sit,* and *stay* when asked, not simply when he feels like it. Reward his obedience. (For detailed information on reward-based training and step-by-step instructions on teaching these commands, please refer to the Appendix.) A reward is anything that he wants and is willing to work for. Food is an obvious

Playing fetch with your dog teaches him to share.

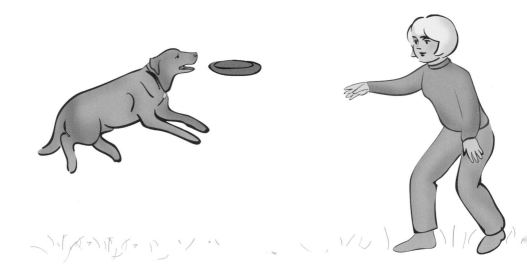

choice, but others are verbal praise and toys. Use low-value rewards (for example, a piece of dry dog food) when training inside the home, and save the higher value rewards, such as cheese, for training outside, where there are more distractions.

You may want to use a "house line" in the home during this training. This is simply a long, lightweight leash, at least 6 feet (1.8 m) long, that is attached to the collar. You use this only when you are at home, to guide him (for example, off the couch) if necessary without having to actually touch him. Once you have so guided your dog, you can then reward him. *Never use a house line to pull a dog toward you for discipline!* Pulling a dog toward you for discipline will scare him and make him perceive you as threatening, which will only serve to deteriorate the relationship that you are trying to build with your dog.

When you first start this training, you may want to show your dog that you have food treats to get him interested, but as you progress each day, switch to hiding the treats in your pocket so that your dog cannot see them. Once he understands a command, wean him off the food treats somewhat by giving him a treat every second time he obeys, and later even less frequently. Don't forget that food is not the only reward!

Take Ownership of Toys and Games

Move all dog toys out of your dog's reach so that he no longer "owns" any of them. Chews and bones can be left out, but they should never be used as toys. You must also play with your dog every day. A few shorter sessions are generally better than one long one, because it keeps both you and your dog focused and interested in doing the work.

In addition, make sure you, not your dog, initiate play. Take

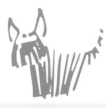

Playing Fetch

It is important to play fetch with your dog, because it teaches him to share. Dogs and owners get enormous enjoyment out of fetch. It is truly an interactive game and can only help strengthen your bond. When he brings the toy back to you, reward using lots of praise and food treats.

out one toy and play only for as long as you want. End the game and put the toy away if he gets overexcited.

Tugging games can be played, but you must win every time. Your dog must release the toy when you ask, and you must reward him after he releases it. Do not release the toy while your dog is holding onto it, because that lets him win. Try to end the game and put the toy away while your dog is still keen on playing. If your dog does not release the item on command, then trade it for a treat when he obeys your command. And if he still doesn't readily release the item, don't play the game, period.

Avoiding Direct Confrontation

Avoid direct confrontation so that your dog knows you are not competing with him. He will then be in a better position to do what you ask. This is particularly important if your dog becomes aggressive toward you (for example, growling when you ask him to do something). By avoiding confrontation, you will also be avoiding a bite.

Discipline Your Dog the Right Way

Never punish your dog after the fact— for example, shouting at him for misbehavior in your absence. He won't associate a past action with your present mood and will likely be confused and fearful of you. If you *do* punish your dog after the fact, he will probably try to calm you down by acting submissively; for example, he may slouch and hang his head and give you a certain look. Many people misread this behavior as "acting guilty."

Also, never use physical punishment or grab your dog by the collar or in any way touch him. It is unnecessary, generally does not work, and can badly damage the relationship between you and your dog.

And without a good relationship, training will be difficult, to say the least. Instead, if you want to show your dog that you are upset with him—while he is behaving badly in your presence— try a time-out. Leave the room for a few minutes, slamming the door behind you. You may also shout before leaving the room, but do not look at him.

Make up with your dog after being upset. Do not hold a grudge. Re-enter the room (if you left it), ask your dog to come and sit, and praise him quietly for doing it. Your dog will clearly know that your anger was caused by his previous behavior. If you are having difficulty getting your dog to move away or off things, such as your furniture, you may want to make use of the house line discussed earlier.

SUMMING UP

In this chapter, we established the importance of taking your dog to the vet for a general health checkup, controlling his behavior, and giving him clear signals that he is not in charge. *You* are in charge, and it's important to demonstrate this whether you are playing with him, teaching him simple commands, or using appropriate discipline.

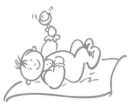

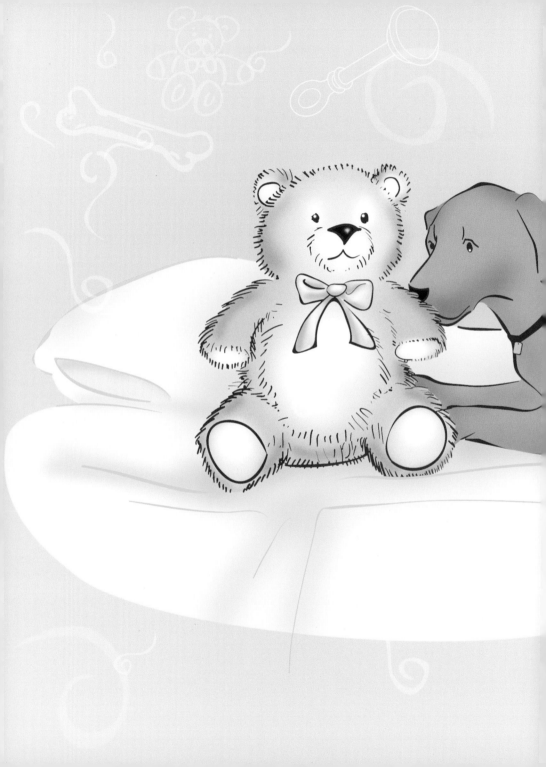

2

THE SECOND TRIMESTER:

Professional Training, Toys, Sounds, and Problem Behaviors

The second trimester of your pregnancy is a time when you can accomplish a great deal with your dog. (This is assuming that no unusual circumstances occur in your pregnancy.) Remember, when we bring pets into our lives, it's a commitment. Or it should be. Dogs expect nothing more of us than a home, food, and kindness. By taking the rather simple steps described in this chapter during and after your pregnancy, you will be returning your pet's devotion in an extraordinarily positive and productive way.

Keeping up status reduction activities is important during the second trimester, and for that matter, throughout your pregnancy and beyond. This activity does not have to be as structured as that described in Chapter 1; rather, it is more of an ongoing reminder to yourself and your pet.

In this chapter, we will cover the widest range of behavior modification. During the second trimester, expectant mommies and daddies will have the most time and motivation for these activities, which include obedience training, not touching baby toys, desensitization to baby sounds, and working to modify problem behaviors.

GET PROFESSIONAL OBEDIENCE TRAINING

In Chapter 1, as part of the status-reduction program, we covered teaching basic commands. For some families, it may be difficult to maintain the necessary consistency of this effort; for others, it may be that their dog is simply not as responsive as they would like. Because of these factors, this is the time to consider professionally guided obedience training. It need not be a highbrow competition course—just a basic program covering the essential commands I described in the last chapter.

A key requirement of this choice is your comfort with how a trainer treats both dogs and owners. I suggest going to a couple of classes and observing them before you make a decision. Modern, reward-based training methods use food, toys, praise, and attention, and these can build on your relationship with your dog—which is not only appropriate, but also fun. In fact, even if you aren't pregnant yet, I strongly recommend professional obedience training anyway. You will never bond more closely with your dog or have more fun with him than

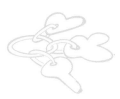

when you take time for this activity.

Your local shelter can refer you to trainers, or you can contact the Association of Pet Dog Trainers (APDT). (Refer to the Appendix for contact information.) APDT members are predominately reward-based trainers who attend an annual conference to further their education in canine behavior and training.

TEACH YOUR DOG ABOUT BABY TOYS

During this time, it is also important to begin teaching your dog not to touch, destroy, or bury baby toys.

You begin, obviously, by selecting toys for your dog that look, feel, and smell different from your baby's toys. This is important, because your dog will find it difficult to differentiate between his own fluffy, squeaky toys and the fluffy, squeaky toys you picked out for your son or daughter.

Ample choices of excellent dog toys are available at your

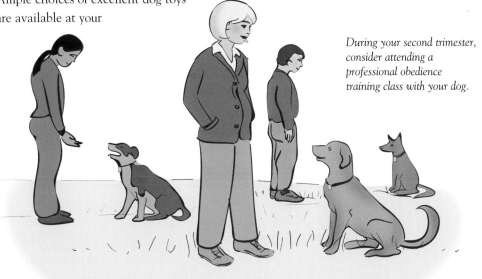

During your second trimester, consider attending a professional obedience training class with your dog.

Toys and Games

Let's reiterate something here about games, because of course that's why you buy toys for your dog. You must be in charge of games—through their initiation, duration, and completion. You are *always* in charge.

neighborhood pet-supply store.

Teaching your dog to ignore your baby's toys is something that can really only be done by you. This process can be tough, simply because similarities between certain dog toys and baby toys cannot be completely avoided. However, it can be accomplished. Here's how: Purchase several toys of the type you plan to have for your baby. Then, spend a few minutes playing with your dog and his favorite toy. When he is fairly excited, take the toy away, but keep it directly in his view. Then, put a couple of baby toys on the floor and toss his into their midst. Encourage him to go get his toy, and then—this is really important—go nuts when he does. If he consistently chooses a baby toy instead and doesn't automatically bring it to you, use a flexi-leash during these exercises, and trade the toy for a treat. The use of a flexi-leash is only to ensure that the dog does not run off and hide the toy. By having him attached to a flexi-leash, you are in control. (This tool is not to be used as a punishment by dragging the dog to you—it is a safety net.)

Repeat this training as often as you can, at least once a week for a month, and slowly increase the number of baby toys each time. It may take many attempts, but persevere. You also may want to consider adding this simple trick to your arsenal: Put a bitter apple spray on the baby toys once a week during training. You can also squirt a little taste of bitter apple spray in your dog's mouth. This will make an even more powerful association that baby's toys taste bad.

If you have a food-obsessed dog, perform the same exercise, but use a food-stuffed toy, such as a marrowbone. Keep practicing until he consistently retrieves his toy and leaves the baby's toys alone.

As your baby becomes older and more mobile, it will be

much more difficult to stop your dog from stealing her toys unless he has done these exercises before. Mobile babies with toys are really exciting and great fun to play with! This is why you should never leave your dog unsupervised with a baby of any age.

DESENSITIZE YOUR DOG TO BABY SOUNDS

If your dog has never been around a baby, it's a very good idea to teach him not to get excited or scared by the crying, screaming, and gurgling he's likely to experience. It's also a very good idea to get yourself prepared because, as a new parent, you may become anxious when your baby cries, and you don't want to communicate your unease to the dog or allow him to misinterpret it.

Teach your dog to differentiate between his toys and baby's toys.

Through a process of desensitization, you must slooooowly condition your dog to sounds that may worry him. You can do this by giving him very small and repeated exposures to these sounds until he treats them as if they are of no consequence. Start by selecting an environment in which your dog feels comfortable—perhaps his favorite room. Also, select a time of day when you are going to be present for at least four hours.

Next, place a CD or tape of baby noises* in your player, and set the volume to the lowest setting. Sit down and relax before turning on the player. (There should be no sound in the room at this time.) Then, put one hand on the volume control and watch your dog closely. Slowly raise the volume until you get

* A CD is available if you are unable to find or create one. See the Resources at the back of the book for ordering information.

the faintest recognition from him—typically, a dog will tilt his head to one side or prick up one or both ears. Once you observe that he is listening to the sounds, leave the volume set at this level for at least three days.

Let the tape play for as long as possible. Twenty-four hours would be ideal, but if this is not possible, then the first exposure must be in excess of four hours. The more the tape is played over the first three days, the better this works. After three or more days, when your dog is no longer taking any notice of the sounds, slowly raise the volume on a daily basis until it is at the level he would normally hear it in this environment. This process varies from dog to dog, but once he is happily listening to the CD at a high level, you can go to the next step, which is moving the player to lots of different locations to expose your dog to the sounds in more natural environments.

This is a desensitization process in which your dog learns to accept the sound without any human or environmental interactions. Thus, don't give him treats for listening to the sounds; just let him relax.

A dog will rarely be agitated or frightened if you are doing the desensitization process correctly. If he does become agitated, then you are going too fast. Slow down. Remember, the more gradually this process is carried out, the more comfortable your dog will be. You should continue to desensitize your dog to baby sounds into the third trimester as well.

MODIFY PROBLEM BEHAVIORS

Some dogs have problem behaviors that must be solved before your baby arrives. Three of the most common are described and addressed here. You can, of course, skip any section that does not apply to your dog, although the information provided may be useful to you in dealing with future behaviors.

I cannot emphasize enough that if you have any doubts about these or other specific problem behaviors, seek professional advice before it's too late!

Aggression

The more a dog is allowed to practice aggression, the better he is at it. A professional trainer should deal with dogs who are truly aggressive toward people and/or dogs and other animals.

Modification Technique

To dogs with a high prey drive, such as those of the herding and hunting breeds, and to dogs who tend to get overexcited with squeaky toys, a baby might not seem much different from prey or a toy. It is therefore important to learn how to direct your dog's drive to something else. Don't let him become obsessed with a ball or a toy that makes a noise—for that matter, don't have squeaky toys in the house. A run in the mornings is a good idea, or a romp in the park might work, because dogs who are regularly exercised make far more relaxed and happy companions who are likely to sleep for the rest of the day. It is also vital to perform the sound desensitization

SECOND TRIMESTER CHECKLIST

1. Get professional obedience training

2. Teach dog about baby toys

3. Desensitize dog to baby sounds

4. Modify problem behaviors

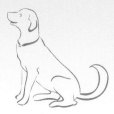

described earlier with these dogs.

Jumping Up

For many people, a dog who jumps up can be very annoying. But it is quite natural for dogs to jump to greet people. Often, they learn that they can get considerable attention by jumping up and grabbing at hands and clothing. Even negative attention such as shouting or pushing the dog away can be rewarding for him. You can train your dog not to jump up, but it is important that all members of your family and all your visitors comply.

Modification Technique

To help your dog learn not to jump up, keep a container of dog treats just outside your front door. When visitors come to your home, they should each put a few treats in their pockets before coming in.

Everyone should ignore all of your dog's attempts to gain attention. Turn your backs, don't move, and pretend he is not even there. No looking, no talking, and no touching! This can be tricky with children aged ten and under, because they have a natural tendency to squeal when a dog jumps up. It is important that they know to not move, and that they keep their hands at their sides and remain quiet.

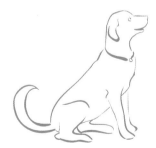

Eventually fed up with being ignored, your dog will sit down or wander off. At this point, you or your visitors can quietly call him forward and ask him to sit. Then, calmly stroke him and give him treats, but only while he stays calm. If he jumps up or becomes overly excited, ignore him again.

Another option for teaching a dog not to jump up is a tie-down—a leash, rope, or cable 2 to 3 feet (0.6 to 0.9 m) long that you attach to an immovable object, like a piece of furniture, or an eyebolt placed in the wall, and to your dog's buckle or flat collar. A tie-down trains your dog to relax and keeps him out of jump-up mischief. In fact, it is a great management tool for a variety of behavioral issues, including:

- barking at the door
- bothering the family at dinner
- jumping up on your bed
- mouthing
- playing too rough

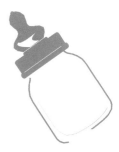

A tie-down should be placed in a fairly busy room in your house, and it should only be used when someone is at home, not when you've gone to work for the day. I can't stress enough that a tie-down is not punishment—it is management. Your dog should be comfortable and have something good to recline on, chew on, and play with while connected to the tie-down. For safety reasons, please do not attach the tie-down to a head collar, choke collar, pinch collar, or any other restricting collars. It should be attached only to flat collars. Make sure that the dog can't drag the piece of furniture around with him or pull the tie-down out of its anchor point.

A tie-down teaches a dog to relax and can help keep him out of mischief.

To set up your tie-down, put the dog on it several times a day for 10 to 15 minutes at a time. You can give him a stuffed chew toy. Then, begin to extend the time the dog is on the tie-down. Vary it so that he doesn't know exactly how long he'll be on it, and he will learn to be patient. If he barks while he's tied, leave the room and return when he's quiet.

Some dogs like to chew pretty much anything they can get their mouth around, including leather or nylon tie-downs. If your dog chews the tie-down, use a cable.

Remember, only use a tie-down when you are at home, and only use it on your dog's flat collar.

Fear of Strangers

Dogs who fear strangers are overbonded to their owners. They follow you around and may suffer from insecurity and destruction problems. Frequently from shelters, these dogs can become too protective of a newborn and make it difficult for parents to get near their infant.

Modification Technique

Stage 1

For one week, divide all your dog's food into ten equal portions for each meal. Feed him in the following manner. First, put him on a lead and touch him all over quickly before offering him the portion of food. Repeat again for each separate portion. Make sure only you or your partner does this for the first week. No other food is to be available for the duration of this program.

Stage 2

For one week, repeat the touching/handling procedures, but now feed most of your dog's food outside the house on walks. Reserve one or two portions of food to be used in the house. When anyone your dog knows and is friendly to enters your home, they should walk straight past the dog without saying a word, go to where the food and toys are, get one portion of

Tie-Downs Versus Tie-Outs

Keep in mind that a tie-down is not a tie-out, which is a cable used to restrain dogs in a yard so that they don't run away. Tie-outs often make dogs aggressive, because the dog can't run away from any perceived threat. I *never* recommend them.

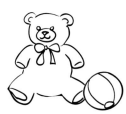

food, and place it on the floor for him to eat. It sometimes helps, if your dog is very friendly toward certain people, to get them to stroke him before giving him the food. They should also engage in toy play in this same location.

Stage 3

Introduce your dog to people whom he does not know quite as well, both inside and outside the house. Begin by chopping up a bit of his favorite food into tiny pieces and putting the pieces into a container. Have a person approach and speak to both of you. Immediately begin feeding your dog pieces of the food, one piece every five seconds, until he is relaxed. Then, have the person take hold of the lead, and if possible, walk him a few paces away before returning to you. This person must hold the lead the entire time. When your dog is relaxed, let the other person stroke and handle him. He should still be fed every five seconds until the food runs out. Repeat this as many times as you can.

SUMMING UP

The second trimester of a pregnancy is a time when you are generally feeling pretty good, with more energy and fewer concerns than during the first or third trimesters. We've covered a wide range of activities you can undertake—the importance of obedience training if needed, desensitization to baby toys and sounds, and modifying specific behavior issues. Problem behaviors are best addressed during this time as well, because they may require more commitment on your part, including professional assistance.

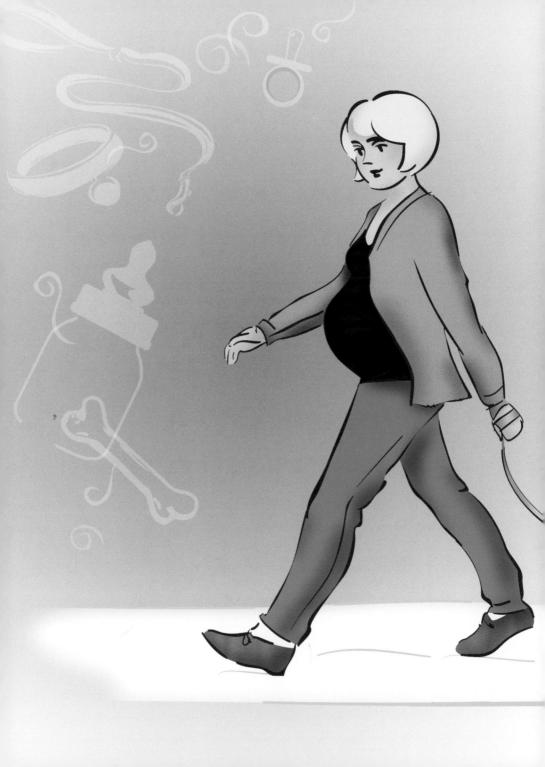

3

THE THIRD TRIMESTER:

Baby Smells, Leash Walking, and Routine Jumble

During your third trimester, it is essential that you continue status-reduction activities, desensitization to baby sounds, and exploration of baby things. Continue refreshing your dog's newly acquired knowledge, and to that, add the activities we cover here.

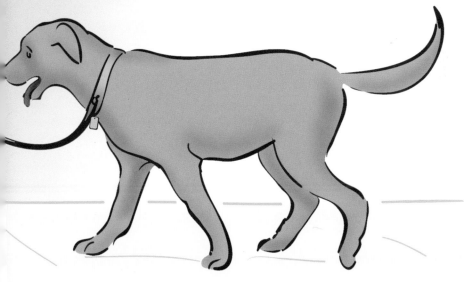

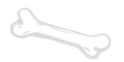

If my son Scott's birth is anything to go by—he was five weeks early, and we didn't have much organized in the way of baby things—it is worth getting a few things ready for baby at the beginning of your third trimester. You don't need to go overboard, but it is a good idea to make somewhere for the baby to sleep, set up a changing area, and store all the clothes everyone is going to give you!

A dog hates change, so it's important to give him the opportunity to check out the nursery and the baby's things before the baby comes. Let him sniff everything, check that no food is around, and just familiarize himself with all this new stuff. Relax and let your dog into the nursery—even feed him in there for a couple of days. Don't make the nursery into a big issue.

If you can't bear the thought of your dog sniffing and drooling all over your baby stuff, then put up a baby gate and

Get your dog used to as many baby smells as possible, including baby powder and lotion.

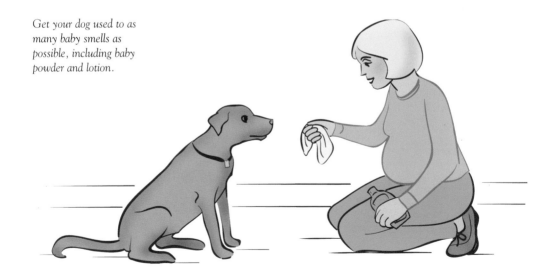

make the nursery out of bounds. Although it is not ideal to restrict your dog's access to baby things, this is not the most important part of the program; your dog and your baby will still develop a relationship. The more access your dog has to baby things and the baby environment, though, the better he will adjust.

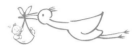

EXPLORE BABY SMELLS

Humans have never really been able to accurately measure a dog's sense of smell. A test was once done in Virginia using one hundred 100-gallon (378.5 l) drums of water. One drop of urine was placed in one drum, and a dog found it in seconds. Not bad, but of course it was a Beagle—the breed to which you may have gathered I am partial.

Think about the impact all the baby smells are going to have on your dog. Let's be honest here—he's not only going to be interested in the baby lotions! I suggest you get your dog used to as many smells as you can, including baby powder, lotion, diaper-rash cream, and so on. Put one smell on a cloth, and leave it in your dog's resting area for a day. Give the dog a day off, and then repeat the procedure with a new scent.

When Scott arrived, I set up a cookie jar full of treats in the nursery for use during diaper changes. The dogs would sit or lie down for cookies while I changed Scott, and thus they lost all interest in the diapers themselves. This became more useful as Scott started to crawl around. When they smelled something, they would dash off to the nursery and wait for us to get there.

To reiterate, it is difficult to measure a dog's sense of smell. Therefore, it is important to allow your pet to become accustomed to the strong- and strange-smelling things that belong to baby.

Plastic Dolls

Some parents believe that using "fake babies" (plastic dolls) will help a dog make the adjustment to a newborn. I emphatically disagree. I believe it is a big mistake to use these dolls. Your dog will know the baby is fake and think of it as a toy, which could be dangerous when your real baby arrives.

WALK NICELY ON LEASH

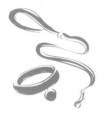

We come now to one of my favorite subjects. In the puppy and adult-dog behavior classes I teach for the Pasadena Humane Society, one of the most rewarding moments for me is seeing the sheer enjoyment owners experience when they are finally able to walk their dogs at their side with a slack leash—that is, the dog is not trying to lead, pulling in all directions, or refusing to move.

Leash walking with your dog is a terrific activity for families, both before and after baby arrives. It's a great exercise for the mommy- and daddy-to-be and just downright fun for the family thereafter. Your relationship with your dog will be greatly enhanced by leash walking, in part because he will associate your baby with fun, well-behaved outings. However, it is *critical* to do this training before baby arrives.

If your dog pulls on the leash, the first step is to fasten the end of the leash to a firm post and then totally ignore any pulling behavior.

The overwhelming majority of dogs do not take naturally to leashes, of course; it is simply not in their nature. Without proper training, they view leashes as a giant distraction. The following section provides general techniques for teaching your dog to walk on a leash, and then some product recommendations that can make the training even easier.

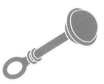

Solving the Leash Problem

These techniques, explained in three stages, are designed for dogs who pull on a leash in all directions, all the time, in an attempt to lead you. I teach them in my classes. Variations on these techniques can be used for other specific issues, but these basic techniques will serve you well in a general way.

Stage One

For about three days, several times each day, put your dog on a leash and collar and simply fasten the end of the leash to a firm post. Allow your dog a radius of about 3 feet (0.9 m) (4 feet [1.2 m] for large dogs), and simply stand next to the post. Totally ignore any pulling behavior. This is easy, because the dog will not be pulling against you. When your dog has stopped pulling for at least ten seconds, tell him how good he is, bend down, and stroke him for at least ten seconds. This procedure ensures that your dog receives no reward at all when he is exerting any pressure on the leash but is rewarded for a fixed period when he is standing correctly. Now stand up straight and repeat the process, rewarding him for ten seconds for every successful ten-second period that he has not leaned or fought against the leash. Keep repeating this until you see a dramatic decrease in the amount of pulling against the leash. Remember that your dog will get tired of pulling before you do.

Stage Two

For about three days, several times each day, attach your dog's leash to his collar and have some small pieces of his daily food allowance either in your pocket or in a small bag. The walk should begin when you attach the leash. Begin by standing still, insisting that your dog stand without exerting any pressure on the leash. When he has been stationary for ten seconds with no pulling, walk forward, keeping the leash slack. Be sure to walk at a pace that *you* want to set. If your dog puts any pressure on the leash at all, *stand still!* Use your leash to insist that your dog return to a position alongside you and that he stand when it is slack. Try to avoid using any commands, because talking to your dog can reinforce the pulling behavior. (We often tend to speak to our dogs most when they are doing something wrong, instead of the other way around—thus reinforcing poor behavior.) Only talk to him when he is not pulling. You are trying to draw attention to the fact that a slack leash results in rewards.

When your dog has remained next to you for around ten

Stage Two of the leash training process involves walking with your dog while carrying small pieces of his daily food allowance in your pocket or a small bag. Use a food treat to reward your dog for not pulling.

seconds, praise him well with your voice for at least ten seconds before moving forward. For every ten paces that you walk and your dog does not exert any pressure on the lead, stop, praise him, and give him a piece of food. The first day that you try this, you may not get very far, but after two or three days, you should see a dramatic decrease in pulling behavior.

Stage Three

From now on, when you walk your dog, you should use a stroller for practice before baby arrives. Before starting out, put some food treats and one or two favorite toys in your pocket. These must be concealed and not shown to your dog before the walk starts. If your dog exerts any pressure on the leash, stand still and don't speak. Use the leash to insist that your dog return to a position alongside you. After a period of at least ten seconds, praise well with your voice before walking forward once again. (Again, it's important to talk to your dog when he's doing something *right*, not wrong.) If your dog is trying to pull you toward something or someone, repeat the above procedure, this time returning to the point at which the dog started pulling. As you get closer to the attraction, your dog's desire to pull will get stronger. You must insist that each time he pulls, he returns to the original starting position before being allowed to try the approach once more. At your discretion, you can allow your dog to meet up with the attraction only when he has walked correctly. When you are walking along, and your dog is not pulling, stop suddenly and produce one of the rewards that you are carrying with you.

Remember that once your dog has learned the correct

Surprise!

Really effective reward-based training involves the element of surprise. When leash training your dog, try to vary the type of reward given, the frequency that it is given, and the amount that is given for the correct walking behavior, so that he doesn't begin to anticipate the treat. Hey, dogs can get bored, too!

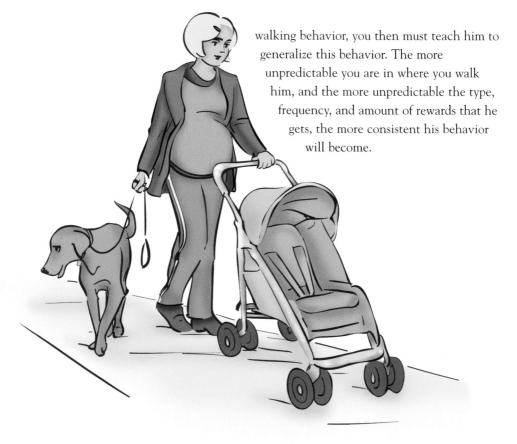

walking behavior, you then must teach him to generalize this behavior. The more unpredictable you are in where you walk him, and the more unpredictable the type, frequency, and amount of rewards that he gets, the more consistent his behavior will become.

In Stage Three of leash training, use a stroller to simulate the walks you will take with your dog once baby arrives.

Leash Products That Work

Two types of products on the market are outstanding for leash training. They are well designed and not harmful to dogs. One is a head halter, and the other is a body harness, to which the leash attaches to the dog's chest.

Head Halter

In my experience, the head halter is ideal for unruly dogs or those who get excitable and lunge when they see other dogs or people. Although it looks like a muzzle, it most definitely is not, because it allows your dog to eat, drink, pant, fetch, and bark while he's wearing it.

The head halter works by applying gentle pressure to the nape of your dog's neck and across his muzzle, in effect mimicking the way a mother dog controls her pup. In action, when walking, it causes your dog to instinctively pull back, not forward, thus helping to eliminate the tendency for leash pulling.

If you plan to train with a head halter, be sure to get the right fit for your dog's size. When you begin working with it, fit the halter carefully, and give your dog treats continuously while he is wearing it. Then, count to 30 and remove the halter. Repeat this at least five times a day for four days before you begin walking. You must desensitize your dog to the head halter and give him a reason to be excited about it. Think about how excited dogs get anticipating a walk when they see a leash; you want to transfer that eager anticipation to the head halter.

Once your dog is desensitized to the head halter, it is time to take him for a walk. Clip the leash to the metal ring under the dog's muzzle, and then pretend you are walking a pony, keeping

THIRD TRIMESTER CHECKLIST

1. Explore baby smells

2. Walk nicely on leash

3. Jumble your dog's routine

a short lead on the leash. As you begin walking—and you should practice with a stroller, keeping the dog to its side—continually praise for good behavior and ignore flip-flopping to either side of the stroller. Try to take as many walks as possible before baby arrives. Be patient. Some dogs just don't understand the head halter right away and take pleasure in manipulating you into stopping.

Body Harness

An alternative to a head halter is a newly designed body harness, which applies humane horse training concepts to teach dogs not to jump, lunge, forge, or pull. Its design employs a front leash-attachment ring at the dog's chest. This allows you to move the lead in different directions to apply gentle body cues, thereby preventing pressure on a dog's throat. Dogs with virtually no leash training at all will start walking with good behavior almost immediately using this harness, although I do recommend using the same start-up procedures as with the head halter.

JUMBLE YOUR DOG'S ROUTINE

Now that your dog knows his place in the household and is used to baby sounds, smells, and supplies, it is vital that you move on to this next stage.

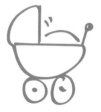

Things are going to be a little hectic when the baby arrives, and your normal routine will be shattered. If your dog has a routine for feeding and exercising, he is likely to react when things don't go quite how he planned. For example, if your dog is fed at 7:00 A.M. every morning and one day the baby needs some 7:00 A.M. attention that takes half an hour, guess who is likely to get slightly frustrated? This frustration can cause your dog to bark, get in the way, or worse, bite one of the parents. If your dog can never anticipate when he is going to be fed or walked, this will not happen. Dogs don't need a routine and actually are far more responsive if they don't have one.

If your dog is currently accustomed to a routine, begin to mix it up a little. Feed and walk him at different times than he is used to. Your life is going to be so hectic for the first few months that you will find it much easier if your dog is not following you everywhere expecting to be fed or walked. Remember to ignore your dog if he is following you around, and after a few days, he will get the message. Trust me—my family lives with two Beagles, and they think that every minute of the day is feeding time!

SUMMING UP

During the third trimester, just as you are winding down to your delivery and getting as much rest as possible, you are also in the winding-down stages with your dog's behavior modification. The tasks I have identified here—exploration of baby smells, leash walking, and routine jumble—are designed to complete your dog's association with a newborn child before her grand arrival!

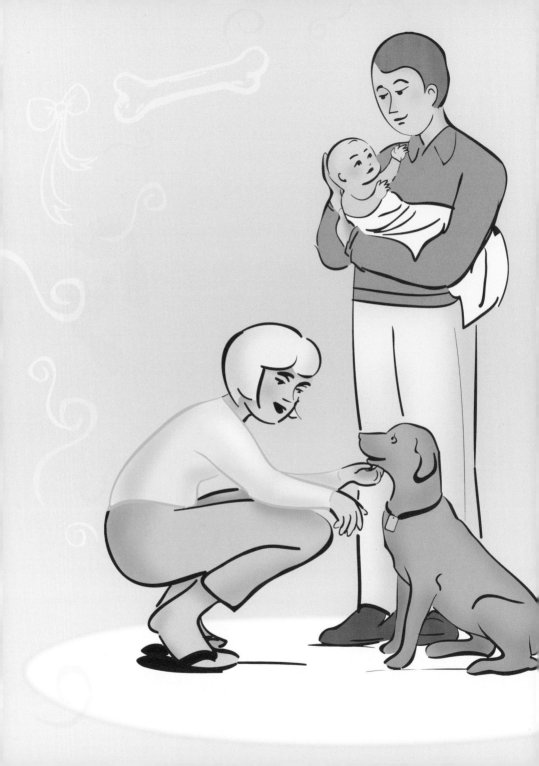

4

iT's TiME!
Hospital Time, Going Home, and Supervision

If your experience is anything like mine (even though Scott was five weeks early), you'll undoubtedly feel as if your pregnancy was 18 months long—as in, won't that time ever get here? Perhaps one of the best benefits of the training you have done up to this point is that it will have filled lots of hours and bonded you even more closely with your dog. More work remains to be done, though. The final touches of your behavior-modification program must be applied during the days before you go to the hospital, the time you are there, the day you come home, and the days and weeks following.

HOSPITAL TIME

When the time comes for you to go to the hospital, make plans for your dog. Is your husband going to come home and feed him, or are your neighbors going to pop in? With Scott coming five weeks early, we had made no plans, and my first few hours of labor were spent trying to sort my dogs out. One could say it was a distraction, but actually it was stressful and something I didn't want to worry about. Make your arrangements in advance, because babies come when they want to!

GOING HOME...AT LAST

When it's time to bring your baby home, it really is quite an event. However, please remember that you have been away from home for a few days, and the dog is going to want to greet you in the worst way. He is not going to be interested in the baby; he is going to be interested in you!

Making Introductions

When you arrive home from the hospital, your dog is going to be overly excited, which may lead to him jumping up. However, he will not jump up if someone else is holding the baby. Make sure your husband, mother, or a friend holds your baby while you reunite with your dog. It will take the anxiety out of the reunion, and you'll be able to act normally around your dog. Spend a few minutes playing with him, then introduce your dog to your baby.

When making the introduction, allow your dog to sniff the baby and lick her feet. It's okay to do this—you have more germs in your mouth than your dog has in his. Talk to your dog in a calm, relaxed manner. Remember to breathe, because you are going to be nervous. Afterward, get him to sit and give him a treat. Repeat this as much as you can, even if you are tired. Every time you, the baby, and the dog are together, invite him over to sniff, and praise him for being so good. Your dog should be rewarded anytime he exhibits calm behavior.

SUPERVISION

Our pets interacted with Scott as an infant quite a lot. The dogs helped me change diapers and entertained him endlessly by retrieving balls that he threw for them. Our cats helped me get him to sleep, soothed him when he was teething, and of course, they were the miracle cure for Scott's hiccups.

Scott and Poppy, the older nervous dog, were inseparable and spent all their waking hours playing fetch. Now, this was

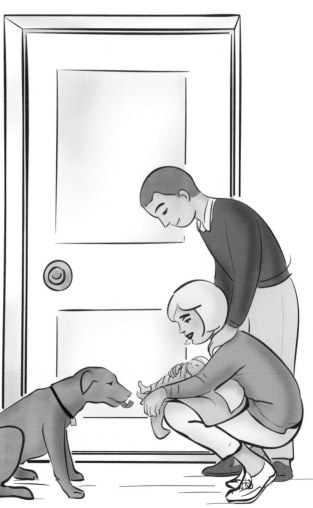

When first introducing your dog to the new baby, allow the dog to lick her feet.

Introducing Your Baby to Your Dog

One of the traditional ways to introduce a newborn to the resident dog is to let him sniff a blanket that your baby has slept on. Certainly there is no harm in doing this, and it will be the first "real" exposure to your baby's specific scent. Do this before you go home, and leave the blanket with your dog overnight. Have someone give him the blanket every day that you are in the hospital. The more exposure he gets to the blanket, the more comfortable he will be with your baby's scent. This may not seem like much, but you've already done most of the preparation!

fetch of a different kind from that played with adults. Sometimes Scott would go out and retrieve the ball; other times, Poppy retrieved. Whoever went after the ball brought it back to the other. However, sometimes Scott picked the ball up, sometimes he just kicked it back, and other times he held it in his mouth!

When I started to potty train Scott, he loved to run around outside with just his diaper on, chasing Caliban. Caliban, a confident young Beagle, often paused to urinate on a bush or even a blade of grass. Scott watched this in amazement, promptly removed his diaper, and lifted his leg right where Caliban had gone. Needless to say, now Scott is completely potty trained and doesn't go outdoors to urinate on bushes—but watching them that summer made me laugh and laugh.

For me, these stories illustrate how much fun and how entertaining babies and dogs can be together, although, of course, this may not be quite the relationship you envision for your child and your dog. The extent of their involvement with each other is a very personal choice and completely up to you. I happen to believe the more involvement, the better. It is so delightful to watch your baby playing happily with your dog. Words really can't describe the feeling.

Still, when he was very young, I never left the dogs alone

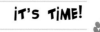
with Scott. All dogs have teeth, and it wouldn't have taken much for ours, as well trained as they were, to let Scott know if he was hurting them. I honestly believe Poppy and Caliban were pretty "bomb proof" while Scott was an infant, but even so, I wasn't prepared to risk my son's well-being to find out.

Scott is seven years old now. He is as close as ever to our pets, and he is quite responsible in their presence. He also likes to go to sleep each night with a dog or a cat, and his choice is a delightful bedtime ritual for us.

Food Refusal

One of the most important supervision issues will occur when your baby begins eating solid food and becomes more mobile. Your dog must know whose food is whose and that snatching food out of your baby's hands, taking it from a table or high chair, and cleaning up the floor below baby's eating area are entirely unacceptable behaviors.

You can get your dog to understand these boundaries with a technique called "food refusal." This can be done before your baby comes home, of course, but you may find it is easier to do after the other training you've accomplished leading up to your baby's arrival.

The training is simple. First, put your dog's favorite treat in your hand and hold it near his nose. When he makes a move toward it, quickly close your hand and use a firmly expressed command, such as "Leave it!" Repeat this at least three or four times, always closing your hand quickly. Never let the dog get the treat.

Many dogs know to sit and wait for you to let them have the treat, so you also must teach a release command, such as "Take it." Then and only then do you leave your hand open and let

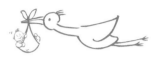

Upping the Ante

You can up the ante in food refusal training by using a higher-value treat. Hot dogs are especially good. To make this variation even more effective, lie down on the floor with your dog and put the high-value treat near his paws. As mentioned earlier, never let him get it until you've given the release command.

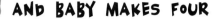
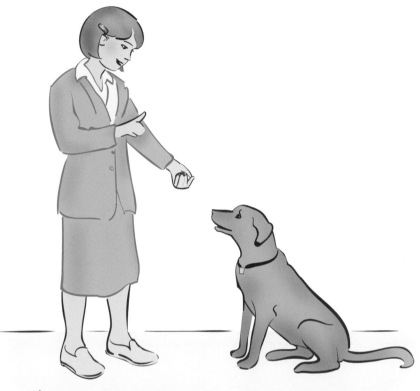

After baby is born, teaching your dog the food refusal technique will help him learn whose food is whose.

your dog take the treat. (The release command can be any word you choose to release your dog at the completion of an exercise.)

A greedy dog—and you undoubtedly know if you have one—may take a bit longer to learn. In addition to this training, put a favorite treat on a table or high chair that would normally be within reach of the dog. Again, when he makes a move, don't let him get the treat. Cover it with your hand and use the *leave it* command. Repeat as often as necessary until Mr. Greedy gets the message.

When teaching your dog the food refusal technique, remember a few things. First, your dog's regular feedings cannot be a part of this training. Don't use his food bowl to teach food refusal, or you'll have a very confused dog on your hands. Second, this is a supervisory issue. If you or your spouse is not in the room to say "Leave it," then a high probability exists that your dog will take food your baby is carrying in his hands or has happened to drop on the floor. You must be there. Third, the key to success here is the same as for any of the other behavioral modifications we've covered so far—practice, practice, practice.

When Baby Is on the Move

Children are of course unsteady when they begin crawling and in the early stages of walking. Their stability and mobility typically advance in fits and starts, with a significant amount of grabbing at this, bumping into that, and falling here, there, and everywhere. In the absence of supervision, this presents risks not only for your baby but also for your dog.

Dogs are very touch sensitive and are therefore quite vulnerable around very young children. You don't want your toddler to fall on your dog or accidentally pull his tail or ears. Long-haired breeds are particularly vulnerable.

If you take a conscientious approach to the training procedures offered in these pages, you will have greatly reduced the possibility that your dog might hurt your child in such circumstances. Still, as I've already noted in this chapter, even the best-trained dogs can be unpredictable. They have teeth, and if hurt, can easily react to the source of their pain. This has the potential to unravel much of the trust you've built up with your dog through previous training.

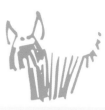

What if You Have a Small Dog?

If you have a small breed dog (or cat), consider putting up a baby gate and raising it off the ground just enough so that your pet can fit underneath. Alternatively, try cutting a small hole in the board so that, if you have a small dog, he can fit through the hole.

Teaching "Over"

You can decrease the risk of your dog reacting poorly when baby is on the move by keeping a close watch for signs of your pet's discomfort and teaching him to exit the room when your baby is crawling or walking. Although many dogs are apt to leave anyway, it is nevertheless easy to show a hesitant dog how to get out of harm's way. Simply fit a 2- or 2 1/2-foot (0.6 or 0.8 m) high board into the doorway to another room, and using a treat or a toy, teach him to go "over" the board and stay in that other room while baby is on the move. Using the board will

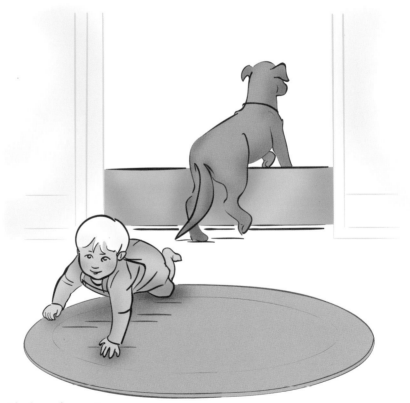

You can decrease the risk of your dog reacting poorly when baby is on the move by teaching him to exit the room.

keep your baby safely confined in the room while allowing your dog to escape.

You can teach your dog to go over the board simply by holding a piece of food under his nose, then throwing it into the other room while saying "Over."

SUMMING UP

In this chapter, we've covered some very specific activities associated with your hospital stay, coming home, and introducing baby and dog. In addition to these activities, I can't stress enough that you should never stop supervising dog and baby when they are in close proximity. Many wonderful opportunities will occur as your child grows past the toddler stage to increase his or her involvement with your dog and to teach gentle handling, proper play, and responsibility. The amount of involvement is up to you. However, I believe the more, the better, because safe interaction is fun, entertaining, and rewarding for every member of the family!

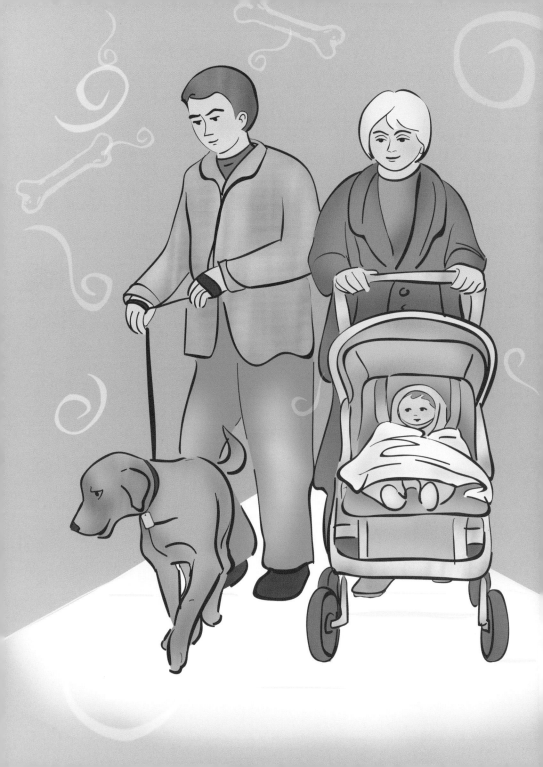

5

iN THEiR OWN WORDS:
Stories of Five Families

During the time I was formalizing and organizing the behavioral-modification procedures that would lead to the writing and publication of this book, I worked directly with several families who owned dogs and were expecting babies. Their experiences became a part of my research and development, and their homes became extensions of the "laboratory" that my own home had become.

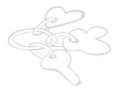

I thought it would be instructive to share their stories with you, so I invited the moms in five of these families to put their experiences into their own words. All the families were successful in addressing specific concerns or problems they had in introducing their newborn into a home where a dog already lived and had assumed the mantle of "firstborn," to whom certain rights and privileges had been granted—chief among them the prerogative to be alarmed about the Invasion of the Dreaded Pink Thing.

RYAN, LISA, AND AIDEN— CALIFORNIA

Ryan is a video editor and Lisa is a stay-at-home mom who runs the family business (editing as well). Lisa worked at home all through her pregnancy. They have two dogs—Ruby, a Corgi mix, and Dutch, a Pit Bull/Labrador mix. Both were three years old when son Aiden came home.

"When Ryan and I found out we were pregnant," writes Lisa, "we were thrilled beyond belief. As my due date approached, I began to get concerned, though. Although Dutch and Ruby are two very friendly dogs, I became incredibly nervous about bringing a new baby into the home.

"We had lots of questions. Would they jump up on us while we held the baby? Would they greet him with love or with anger? How could we make sure Dutch and Ruby would not feel jealous or left out? Would they be good dogs to have in the home with a newborn, and later with an older baby? How would they react to our son's cries? How would we introduce the dogs to Aiden?

"We consulted Penny, who gave us a CD of her son crying (but wouldn't listen to it with us…a true mom!) and taught us how to introduce the noise to the dogs and teach them to ignore the cries. She gave us some guidelines to follow to get the dogs prepared. For example, they started sleeping in the living room—not in our bed.

"Penny continued to encourage me that it would be okay. And she was right. We did exactly what she said when we brought Aiden home for the first time. I made sure that I went in first and said hello to Dutch and Ruby before they met him. They immediately loved Aiden. And because we had desensitized them to his noises, they were great when he cried—they reacted, but calmly. Dutch and Ruby were very gentle with him. Aiden is five months old now, and he and the dogs interact beautifully.

"I'm certain that without doing this training before bringing Aiden home, the entire experience would have been stressful and chaotic instead of the happy, exciting time it was!"

MICHELE, BRIAN, AND BRANT— CALIFORNIA

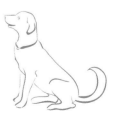

Michele is a homemaker and Brian is an engineer. Michele was at home throughout her pregnancy with their son, Brant. The couple owns Cocoa, a Cattle Dog/Chow mixed breed who is now

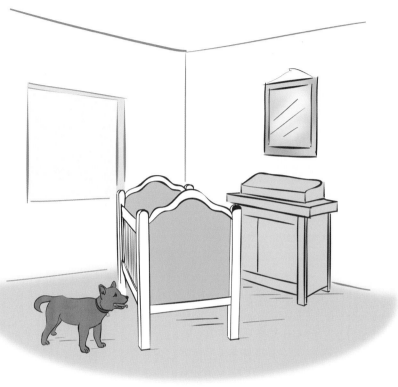

Cocoa was allowed to roam inside the baby's room as more baby furniture began to appear.

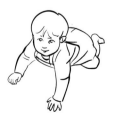

two years old.

"Soon after we adopted Cocoa, we enrolled her in a general dog training class at the Pasadena Humane Society. Four months prior to Brant's birth, we did a two-part Baby–Dog Introduction training.

"Cocoa's behavior prior to the baby–dog training was fairly good and very energetic. She loved to be included in our daily events, so we allowed her to be with us as much as possible. We

would usually walk her daily, as well as play fetch-the-tennis-ball with her. She is, however, a stubborn dog and is also very protective of us and of our home. In the past, she had a habit of jumping up on us and "play nipping." She is also very leery of strangers and would possibly try to bite an intruder.

"We were somewhat wary of Cocoa's ability to "succeed" in being a well-mannered, gentle dog around our baby. We did not want her to fail—by showing aggression toward the baby—or to feel forgotten or jealous once we brought Brant home. My husband and I agreed prior to his birth that if Cocoa showed aggression toward our son—biting or growling, for example—then we would need to place our dog with another family. We truly did not want this scenario to result, as we are very close to our dog. So we sought out Penny to work with Cocoa and us on an individual basis to come up with a specific training plan. We also wanted accurate information concerning how to introduce the family dog to a baby and safety tips to follow thereafter.

"The training included sensory desensitization with visual, olfactory, and audio stimuli exercises. For example, I applied various baby products, one at a time, to a clean rag and then would place it on Cocoa's bed for a day. Cocoa would briefly sniff the rag and even sleep on top of it, not appearing to be that interested in the new smells. She was allowed to roam inside the baby's room as more baby things and furniture began to appear. Cocoa seemed to be somewhat more interested in the baby's room, as she exhibits sight-dog tendencies and probably noticed the new things. Lastly, we played a CD with sounds of a baby crying and fussing. First, we adjusted the volume of the CD player so that the sound was barely audible to the human ear. Every couple of days we

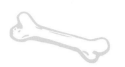

raised the volume until it was finally rather loud. We could only stand this exercise for a couple of hours per day for two to three weeks! Cocoa seemed to be interested in this new crying sound in the beginning of the exercise and later would go outside to get away from the noise.

"The greatest challenge for us with Cocoa was leash pulling. For a while after Brant's birth, two of us needed to walk her, with one of us handling the dog and the other carrying our son. For the first three months after my son was born, I feared that if I walked Cocoa alone with Brant, I might fall or not be able to effectively control Cocoa. More recently, I have become more comfortable walking Cocoa while I have Brant strapped to me in a baby carrier. We have immensely enjoyed our walks since the training.

"The greatest rewards include knowing that we can trust Cocoa around our son in a supervised manner, and how they seem to really like each other. Brant often watches Cocoa (it's great entertainment for him) or reaches out to touch her. Cocoa allows this and is very gentle with Brant. Our dog has always enjoyed "pack moments." She will often lie next to us on the carpet and lick his hands or feet while we're holding him on our lap. She seems to understand that her place in the pack is below Brant but that she is still important. Sometimes, when our son is having a fussy period, Cocoa has a look of concern on her face in her own kind of doggy way. She will sit with us until everything seems better.

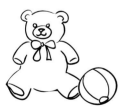

"Another area of great satisfaction is the knowledge that Cocoa also seems happy with the new addition to the family. At first, we were very cautious and kept Cocoa behind a baby gate in the kitchen. She would watch us in the dining room

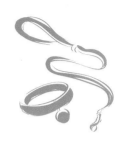
with a sad look on her face. Three days after we brought our baby home, the gate came down and we allowed her to sniff our son. Gradually, we saw how Cocoa understood that the baby was to be respected and that she seemed relatively content. We have tried to maintain some sort of routine for Cocoa to let her know that we still care about her. This includes activities such as playing her favorite game of tennis ball with her, hiking on trails near our home, and taking neighborhood walks.

"Actively preparing our dog for Brant's arrival has given us the knowledge and tools for a successful dog–baby introduction and nurturing a good relationship with Cocoa. We are thrilled that everything has worked out so well!"

GILLAN, GREG, AND AXEL—CALIFORNIA

Gillan is a realtor and Greg a general contractor. She worked 20 to 30 hours per week prior to the birth of their son, Axel. The family owns two dogs—Bella, a Chow and Border Collie mix, and Monty, a Labrador and Rottweiler mix. They were nine and seven years old, respectively, when Axel came home.

"My initial fear was that Bella would withdraw from the family and become more aggressive once we brought Axel home. I had far fewer concerns about Monty, who is mellower.

"There is a lot to recommend about training your dog for the arrival of a baby. For us, using a baby crying tape was extremely helpful. It actually prepared all of us, including the

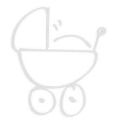

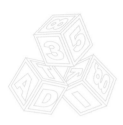

cats, for what was coming. Bella and Monty were both anxious at first, as the sound of crying was completely foreign to them. I played it very low to start and gradually increased the volume over several weeks. The dogs became more relaxed and eventually didn't even seem to notice the new noise.

"When Axel was born, Greg brought home blankets and diapers and let the dogs get used to the baby's scent before the baby came home. This was another success. When Axel finally came home, the dogs sniffed him and then went about their day.

"Our son is 14 months old now, and he interacts beautifully with Monty, snuggling up to him like a large stuffed animal. Bella is very good around him, too, though I limit physical contact out of respect for her boundaries. While she likes to keep to herself, she is also protective of him."

BILL, GINGER, AND ELIZABETH HOPE— CALIFORNIA

Both Ginger and Bill are clinical psychologists. Ginger worked until the final two weeks of her pregnancy. The family dog is Shorty, a Beagle and Dachshund mix, who was approximately eight years old at the time of Elizabeth's birth.

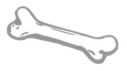

"Our hope was that we could learn to deal with Shorty's excitability and protectiveness around children. He would bark and lunge at children when we walked him. Thus, we were quite concerned about how he'd behave around our infant. Our

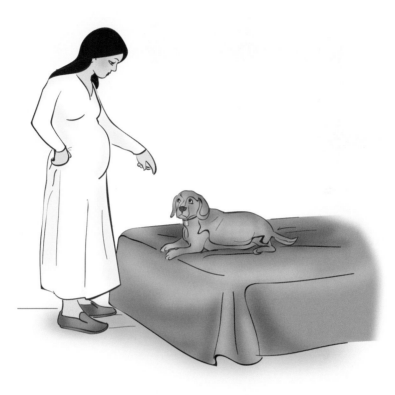

biggest fear was that he would be jealous of Elizabeth and would act out aggressively.

"When we first consulted Penny, the reality of our 'only child,' Shorty, needing to adjust to a little sister was looming in the not-so-distant future. We couldn't bear to think of the potential for a dangerous situation, because Shorty had been somewhat aggressive with other children in the past. We knew

Part of Shorty's status reduction plan was not allowing him access to the bed.

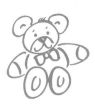

we needed to help him be prepared for this big transition in all our lives.

"When we met, we were told that Shorty was a good candidate for a status-reduction program. For him, that entailed not letting him sleep on our bed anymore, not getting on our couch, and not getting anything for free. This meant that Shorty had to sit and shake hands to get his dinner and go outside. The sitting and shaking hands part was okay, but not letting him on the bed was extremely difficult. For years, he had been sleeping there while we were at work. It was really his domain. Telling him he had to get off the bed was something that really made no sense at all to him.

"Penny recommended we keep our bedroom doors closed so that Shorty would not have access to the bed. We did that, and yet sometimes he would still get in the room if we forgot to close the door right away. Shorty would come in immediately and jump up to his favorite spot. Penny recommended that we yell loudly for him to get off the bed but not look directly at him while yelling. We did this for several months, and he eventually, though reluctantly, got the message. Shorty no longer considers our bed to be his domain. He also does not get on the couch unless he is invited up.

"For the most part, Shorty is very good with Elizabeth and has not displayed any aggression toward her. Shorty only likes to be in the same room when we are with her. He is a much better behaved and happier dog. He is so much calmer!"

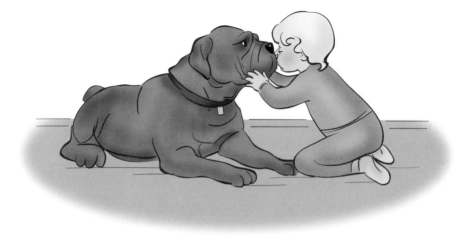

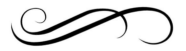

Thunder has been trained to be gentle and loving with Tessa.

JENNIFER, BRENT, AND TESSA— CALIFORNIA

Brent works full time as a director of digital strategies for a record management company, and Jennifer works part time from home in nonprofit management. She was not working when their puppy was new to the home, during her last month of pregnancy with daughter Tessa.

"Our dog, Thunder, is an English Mastiff. He is 18 months old now. We began training him for the arrival of our new baby when he was four months old. He is, and has always been, a

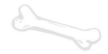

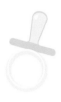

very sweet, lovable large dog who needs a lot of attention. Therein was the challenge: He was a bit pushy in order to get the attention he craved.

"We had had a very bad experience with a previous dog, Gryphon, a Pit Bull terrier. Another dog who was off leash charged at him. I tried to get Gryphon to release the other dog, but he would not, and the other dog was killed. As a result, we wanted to be certain that we could control Thunder in almost any situation, but especially with a newborn in the house. It was critical that he be 'baby trained' and obedient.

"We enrolled in Penny's behavior training class for puppies. The eight-week session went through basic commands (*sit, down, stay*), through more challenging commands such as *fetch, come*, and *heel*. We also worked on Thunder's attention-seeking and 'pushy' behavior. He was very responsive to most of the lessons, but the most effective was the attention-seeking training. He had absolutely hated being ignored and learned to calm down immediately.

"We knew Thunder was a sweet dog the moment we chose him, but the impact of appropriate training has made the day-to-day interaction with him much more positive and valuable. He is more involved in our family activities because he is well behaved and follows instructions.

"Thunder and Tessa, now 17 months, are virtually inseparable. He is the first thing Tessa wants to see in the morning and the last before she goes to bed. This is a testament to how loving, gentle, and wonderful Thunder is to her. He rarely goes near her toys, although some wooden ones I think are hard for him to resist. He doesn't knock her over and is very careful when moving around her. Tessa has gone through a few

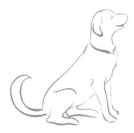

stages of not being completely gentle with Thunder, and he just calmly looks at her with his big brown eyes and waits for what is next. Tessa can give Thunder his treats, food, and toys, and he ever so gently takes them from her little hand. Tessa frequently will go up to Thunder when he is relaxing and kiss him or hug him. His response is to lick her face or head. They are wonderful friends and playmates. We could not have asked for a better dog. Thunder was a sweet dog to begin with, but the training we went through made him a fantastic playmate for Tessa (and the rest of the family)!"

SUMMING UP

Although it is certainly instructive to read these experiences, I recognize that not all families are going to have the time, the budget, or the inclination to engage a professional trainer to help them prepare a dog for the arrival of a newborn, as these five families did. That's why the techniques and tips I gave them are laid out in this book for you. Desensitization to baby sounds, status-reduction, teaching a dog not to touch baby toys, jumping up issues—all that and many more training opportunities are covered in these pages. I very much encourage you to pursue them on your own. If you truly love your dog and want him to adapt to baby easily, then following the principles offered here will be one of your most rewarding experiences.

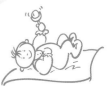

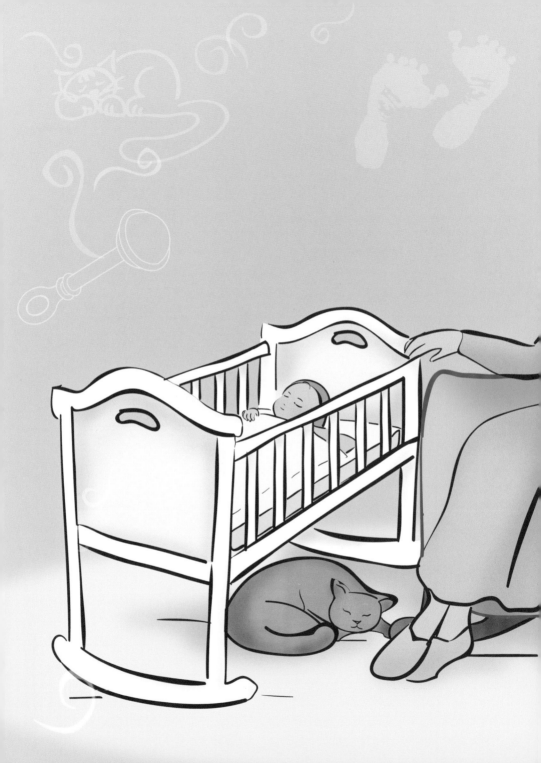

6

OTHER FOUR-LEGGED FRIENDS:

Cats

Ah, cats.

Chances are, if you have a dog, you might also have another four-legged friend—a cat. And if you thought by this point that I was giving cats short shrift, you're been partly right—although it has nothing to do with a lack of affection, experience, or concern for their well-being when baby comes home. The truth is that you have far less to do when it comes to preparing cats for a new baby. Why? Because compared to dogs, cats are sooo much easier.

THE TRUTH ABOUT CATS

Cats are very rarely aggressive and indeed are likely to be afraid of babies. In the scheme of things, dealing with a baby is probably item number 233 on a cat's List of Things to Do Today. They would rather just get out of the way, actually.

It is not true that cats like to "steal a baby's breath," as the old wives' tale goes. It is true that they like a cozy place to sleep, and cribs with babies in them are a favorite. That's okay, as long as you are present. If you must be out of the baby's room, though, you can put a cat tent over the crib. These are available in baby stores.

It is not okay for your cat to knead your baby, which is why you should keep his claws trimmed—trimmed, not removed! It is also not okay for him to groom your baby with his tongue (although it is okay for him to groom himself around baby, because it means he is relaxed and happy). If he does these things, remove him from the room. He'll get the idea.

ADAPTING TO CHANGE

Cats are less adaptable to change than are dogs. Even the slightest change in a household can affect them. This is particularly true of shy cats, those apt to become anxious and hide when you have visitors. If you have a shy cat, try using Rescue Remedy, a completely natural herbal product available in health food stores. For two to three weeks before baby comes home, and for two to three weeks after, give your cat three drops morning and night. I can no offer no scientific basis for this claim, only my own experience, but I have seen cats become far less anxious after being treated with Rescue Remedy.

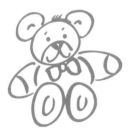

HEALTH CONCERNS

A more serious concern with our feline friends is a parasite

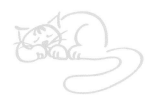

called *Toxoplasma gondii*, which causes toxoplasmosis, a disease that can be transmitted from cats to humans. The medical profession rightly believes that this parasite can be dangerous to pregnant women, although I am far less confident in the judgment of some doctors that the best solution to this *potential* problem is putting cats up for adoption.

Toxoplasmosis is shed through cat feces. It could be transmitted to you if you were to come into contact with feces. The obvious solution is to wear disposable rubber gloves when you empty the litter box—or better still, get your spouse to do it!

A couple of additional tips about litter box management are in order. Buy the cheapest brand of litter available. Cats are not at all concerned about the elegance of this experience. Instead of putting 3 inches (7.6 cm) of the stuff in the box, as so many people do, put in half an inch (1.3 cm). It's all that's necessary. In this way, you can dispose of the litter on a daily basis without it becoming either a cost or a potential sanitary issue. Follow these procedures, along with the use of rubber gloves and/or my recommended "spousal poop patrol," and you should have no problem with toxoplasmosis.

Did You Know?

Cats are very rarely aggressive and are likely to be afraid of babies.

HELPFUL HINTS

Here are some helpful hints to keep your cat happy and healthy, while at the same time keeping your baby safe:

- Get the same vet check as you would for your dog before baby comes home.
- Let your cat explore your baby's things so that he becomes familiar with them.
- Keep your cat's nails trimmed short for safety and also to preserve your furniture. Cats scratch furniture to shed the cuticle on the outside of their claws. If the

nails are trimmed regularly, they won't need to do this. Using human or cat nail clippers, trim the nails to just above the red vein, which is easy to see in a cat's claw. There is no reason to declaw a cat when the baby comes; not only is the practice inhumane, it is also illegal in many parts of the world.

- Help your cat stay clean with regular brushing and flea treatment (topical preparations are more effective than collars), and change his litter box daily.

Cats and babies can get along quite well together.

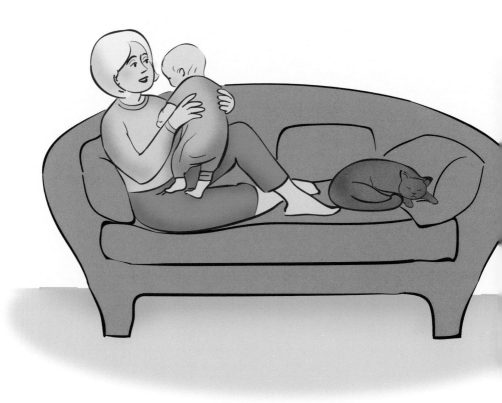

- Keep your crawling infant out of your cat's reach, which is not likely to be very hard, because your cat would rather be out of baby's reach anyway.
- Never force a cat into a situation with a child—as, for example, "Wouldn't it be just adorable if we took a picture of Bobby Junior holding Fluffy?" Not a good idea.

SUMMING UP

Cats are rarely aggressive toward a newborn, and by giving your furry friend an opportunity to leave the situation rather than forcing contact, he will come around in his own time. In short, a cat will probably be the least of your concerns, pet-wise or otherwise, when your baby comes home!

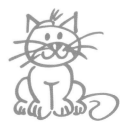

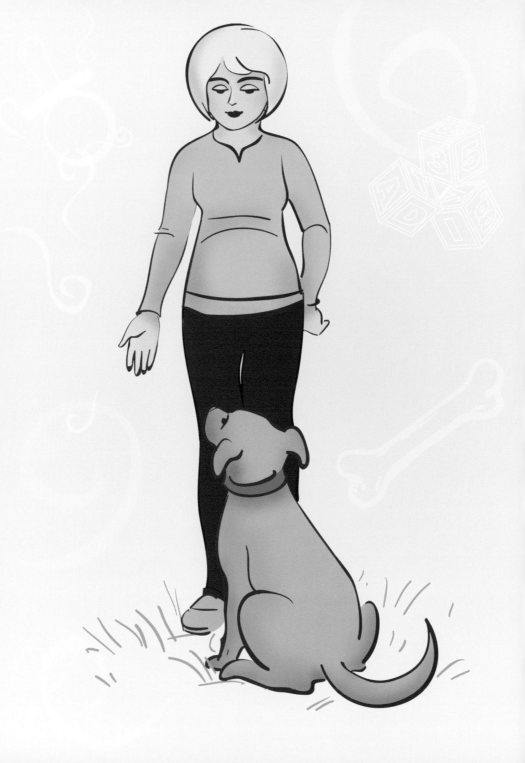

ᐧAPPENDIX:

Positive Training and Basic Commands

Throughout this book, I have referenced four common commands—*sit, down, come,* and *stay*—that your dog should obey even before you began reading this book, but especially as a prelude to preparing him for the arrival of your baby. Perhaps, however, your dog has mastered only a couple of them, or none. *Tsk, tsk, tsk.*

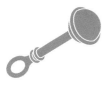

As a bonus to you, dear reader, this chapter will teach you how to teach your dog these basic behaviors. Now, don't be alarmed. The methods you'll learn here are not the type used for competition training; they are simply for regular, everyday obedience. You should find them fun and easy to accomplish.

POSITIVE TRAINING

The key to any training is a good relationship with your dog, one in which he is rewarded for doing exactly what you want him to do. Rewards aren't limited to food—they can be toys, attention, smiles, games of fetch, and the freedom to run. The important thing is that dogs always should be rewarded for doing a behavior correctly; otherwise, there's not much in it for them. Some people misinterpret this as bribing a dog to elicit the correct behavior. It is not bribery; the point of any training is to build a relationship with your dog that is enjoyable for both of you.

Discover What Your Dog Likes

The positive training process begins with making notes about what your dog really likes. Start by listing five different foods that he loves. Ideally, his regular dog food should be on that list. A few words about that: If your dog doesn't love his food and eat it happily, change to another brand. Why? Could it be that you have been "encouraging" him to eat by putting a little cottage cheese, chicken broth, bits of bacon, or similar enhancements in his food? My friend, you are being manipulated. Although there is little wrong with feeding human-grade food to dogs—chocolate, raisins, and onions are serious exceptions that can harm them—yours is obviously

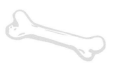

holding out for something other than just his dog food, and you are giving in. Eventually, this behavior must stop. Remember, you are in charge of the relationship. Heed the story of an Akita who, by the time he was five years old, had managed to train his owners to cook five chickens for him every day! Get the picture? Find a regular dog food that your dog loves and will work for as a reward. Scores of dog food brands are on the market; one of them will be his passion. You can still have human-food treats on your favorites list for training time or special occasions, but they can no longer be part of his regular daily diet.

Next, list five toys or games your dog loves, five different places that he likes to go, and five different touches he enjoys. Recognizing what touches he likes is simple; you'll be able to tell that your dog likes certain kinds of touch if he is relaxed and feels pliable under your fingertips, and if sometimes he would rather be close to you than across the room. Just be observant. Our Poppy adores having the top of her nose kissed, while her partner Beagle, Caliban, loves having his ears scratched.

Speak "Dog"

Let us also briefly consider another, little understood point before we get to the basic behavior training. Dogs do not speak English. They do not understand any human languages or words. They speak "Dog"—that is, they respond primarily to sounds. In their interactions with us, they react to the sounds we teach them, as well as to our tone of voice, our smiles, and other physical gestures. As human beings, we tend to ascribe human-type abilities and personalities to our pets. But at the

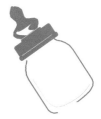

end of the day, they are still dogs, and in their training, they learn by the *sounds and rewards* you associate with specific behaviors.

Frankly, many people talk too much to their dogs anyway. Don't get me wrong. It is great to talk to your dogs, but when you find yourself constantly repeating a command for a behavior, you have a problem. Don't assume that repeating (or yelling) the same command over and over will make your dog obey. In fact, the reverse will occur—your dog will tune you out, and he won't understand why you're yelling at him.

BASIC TRAINING

It is important to have a dog who listens to you and performs basic commands when you ask. This section provides you with the tools you need to teach your dog some basic commands, like *sit*, *down*, and *stay*, and most importantly, to come when called.

In any kind of obedience training, try not to manipulate your dog into a position. Instead, get him to "choose" it. You do this by offering a reward, such as treats, praise, or petting to lure him into position. This has a much more powerful impact, and your dog will learn better. Once your dog understands what you want, and you are able to communicate your wishes, you can use the top rewards (those he likes best) intermittently, as a surprise.

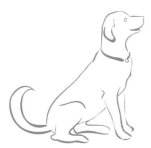

Sit (Getting Your Dog's Rear End on the Ground)

Before teaching this command, first divide your dog's daily food into ten portions; this gives you ten training opportunities.

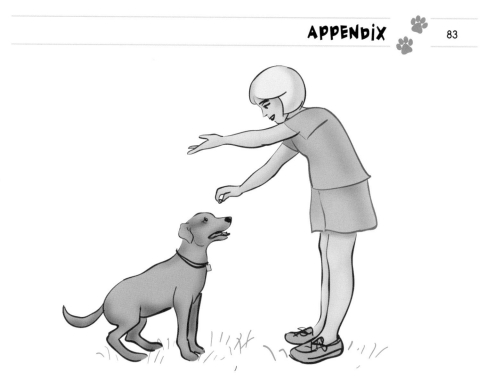

Have your dog sit at various times throughout the day, so that he earns each portion of food. If you don't have time for ten training opportunities, do as many as you can. A minimum of four should be possible, even for the busiest of families.

When teaching the sit command, the first step is to hold a piece of kibble in front of you and raise it above your dog's head.

How to Teach Sit

1. Hold a piece of kibble in front of you, and raise it above your dog's head. Most dogs will follow the trajectory of the food and automatically sit.

2. Call him by name to get his attention, as in "Poppy!" Once your dog looks at you, give him the kibble.

3. Next, use a hand signal that will work for you and say "Sit!" once. (I use a clenched fist in front of my waist, while other people point to the dog's rear end. A hand

signal can be anything you want, as long as it is consistent.) As soon as your dog's rear end hits the ground, hand-feed the portion of food. Simultaneously, smile lavishly and praise your dog. Try not to repeat the command, because the dog will start to tune you out.

Once you feel that your dog has mastered this behavior, choose different locations around your house and yard in which to practice. The goal is to teach your dog to perform the *Sit* anywhere, so go to more and more distracting environments as he gets better. When you are in a really distracting place for your dog, use a higher value treat, and remember to always end on a positive note of praise.

Down (Getting Your Dog to Lie in the Sphinx Position)

Again, divide your dog's daily ration of food into ten portions and follow virtually the same training schedule as outlined for teaching the *sit* command.

How to Teach Down

1. Have your dog sit.
2. Hold one portion of food in your hand just below his nose.
3. Move your hand toward the floor; keep his attention on the food, but do not allow him to take it.

Use a treat to lure your dog into the down *position.*

4. Eventually, your dog will become tired of holding his head

down and will begin to lie down to get more comfortable. As soon as he starts to lie down, say "Down," and give him the reward and praise him when he reaches the correct position.

Stay (Getting Your Dog to Remain in Position—*Sit* or *Down*—Until Released)

The *stay* can be tricky. The traditional way of teaching it— not a good way, in my opinion—was to have a dog sit or down, say "Stay," and walk slowly away. If the dog got up or broke the stay, you rushed back, repositioned him, and repeated the process. Normally, you walked away backward—not something humans typically do—and became anxious because you were worried that the dog would get up. From the dog's point of view, the whole situation seemed strange, because his owner was behaving nervously. Naturally, the dog would break his *stay*.

Also, in the old way, you called your dog out of a *stay*—you told the dog to stay, walked some distance away, and then turned and called the dog back to you. I don't think this is a good idea, because some very sensitive dogs naturally break as soon as eye contact is made, which of course is not what you want at all.

How to Teach Stay

I teach *stay* differently. First, putting cart before horse, all dogs should be taught that they will be released from a *stay*. In this way, the training will really take. Specifically, you must always go back to release your dog so that you can reward him for being so clever. Choose a release command like "Okay" or

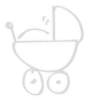

"Free" when you want your dog to get up. Now, here are all the steps:

1. Attach a leash to your dog's collar, and tie the leash to an immovable object.
2. Place ten treats about ten paces away.
3. Have your dog sit or lie down, and then tell him "Stay."
4. Walk away from him to the treats in a calm, unemotional manner.
5. Pick up a treat and return to your dog. If he remains in the *sit* or *down* with a slack leash, give him the treat. Praise, smile, and tell your dog how great he is.
6. If your dog gets up as you are walking toward him with the treat, do not give it to him. Put him back into a *sit* or *down*, tell him to stay, and repeat steps 4 and 5.
7. Repeat this process until all treats are gone.
8. When you are finished, calmly return to your dog, unclip the leash, and use your release word to finish the exercise.

Repeat this exercise four times per day.

After a couple of days of being tethered, fake your dog out by pretending to tie him up. Practice as if he thinks he is tied.

Give your dog a treat if he exhibits a calm, patient stay.

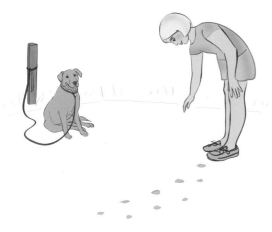

Once you feel your dog really understands what is going on, you can start going into other rooms in the house, leaving him in a *stay*. If your dog breaks the *stay*, you are moving too fast. Go back to tying him again. Your dog will learn that you will come back—but remember, do not exhibit any anxiety in this training!

Come (Getting Your Dog to Stop What He Is Doing and Come Back to You)

This is one of the most beneficial behaviors you can teach your dog. Being able to call him back to you ensures that he can be let off leash safely. Using your dog's absolute favorite treats is essential for this training.

How to Teach Come

1. Begin in your house. Start calling your dog enthusiastically, and be sure that you have a good reward ready when he reaches you. Praise him and give him his reward when he comes to you, and let him know how great he is.

2. Do the same thing in your backyard. Gradually build up the distance, practicing frequently throughout the day. Reward him well each time until he is rushing to you at top speed whenever you call him, even if he is busy doing something else.

3. Play hide-and-seek in your house and yard. Have someone hold your dog while you go off and hide. Call your dog, and reward him for finding you. Not only is this great fun, but dogs also love that we get so excited when they come to us.

Now that you have taught your dog to come to you in an easy, nondistracting environment, go out into the real world, around big distractions—dogs, squirrels, and cats, for example. If you have performed the first three steps correctly, your dog will love coming to you, regardless of the distraction.

1. Take your dog on a long line to a quiet area outside. When he is looking away from you, call him using the

same words that you used in the first three steps. Reward him for coming back to you. Speed up the return by running backward a bit. Reward him when he gets to you.

2. When he responds readily to your call in a quiet outside area, practice in slightly more distracting places. He must be really coming to you before you change to a new location. Use the light line to encourage him to return if he doesn't come right away.

As in all things, practice makes perfect. Practice this behavior diligently, because teaching your dog to come back to you will go a long way toward ensuring his safety and your peace of mind.

Use a long line to teach your dog to come in an outdoor environment.

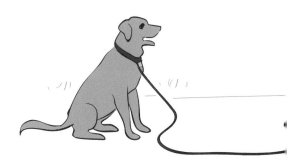

SUMMING UP

Giving your dog the ability to sit, down, stay, and come enhances his preparation for the great change coming to your life in a significant way. Many of the other behaviors your dog must learn before your newborn comes home—not touching baby toys, leash walking, status-reduction training, and others—are made that much easier if your dog responds easily and happily to the basic behaviors covered here. Teaching these commands to your dog is well worth your time, doesn't require a lot of time, and is fun for both of you.

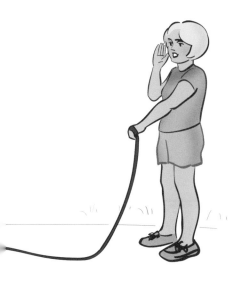

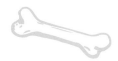

RESOURCES

Below are some wonderful resources for pet owners, some of which I referred to in the book, as well as links to websites of interest for all who care about the welfare of animals.

ASSOCIATIONS

Association of Pet Dog Trainers
150 Executive Center Drive Box 35
Greenville, SC 29615150 Executive
Center Drive Box 35
Telephone: 1-800-PET-DOGS
Fax: 1-864-331-0767
E-mail: information@apdt.com
www.apdt.com

This is a professional organization for dog trainers, with useful information for dog owners, too. Their website offers a complete listing of trainers around the world

Pasadena Humane Society & SPCA
361 S. Raymond Avenue
Pasadena, CA 91105
Telephone: (626) 792-7151
Fax: 626-792-3810
www.phsspca.org

My home away from home, included here not only because it's such a fabulous place, but also because on their website, on the "Links" page, you will find an extraordinary array of website addresses for national and international animal welfare organizations.

SHELTERS AND RESCUE ORGANIZATIONS

As I noted in the Introduction, not all dogs or cats are born to live with babies. Some simply cannot be trained, and if this is your situation, it is best for all concerned that your pet be rehomed. I urge you to contact the humane society organization in your community.

American Humane Association (AHA)
63 Inverness Drive East
Englewood, CO 80112
Telephone: (303) 792-9900
Fax: (303) 792-5333
www.americanhumane.org

American Society for the
Prevention of Cruelty to Animals
(ASPCA)
424 E. 92nd Street
New York, NY 10128-6804
Telephone: (212) 876-7700
www.aspca.org

Royal Society for the Prevention of
Cruelty to Animals (RSPCA)
Telephone: 0870 3335 999
Fax: 0870 7530 284
www.rspca.org.uk

The Humane Society of the United
States (HSUS)
2100 L Street, NW
Washington DC 20037
Telephone: (202) 452-1100
www.hsus.org

Gentle Leader® Head Collar
Premier Pet Products
14201 Sommerville Court
Midlothian, VA 23113
Telephone: 888.640.8840
Fax: 800.795.5930
E-mail: info@premier.com
www.gentleleader.com

SENSE-ation™ Harness
29460 Union City Blvd.
Union City, CA 94587
Telephone: (866) 305-6145
Fax: 510-487-2928
www.softouchconcepts.com

PRODUCTS

Baby Sound Compact Discs &
Tapes
Sound Good CD—Babies (by Terry
Ryan)
1-800-776-2665
www.dogwise.com

INDEX

ACKNOWLEDGEMENTS

I would like to express special thanks to my son, Scott, and our family's "four-legged children," Poppy, Caliban, Chenega, and Kenaitze, without whom none of this would have been possible; to Gillian Abercrombie and Greg Frame, Ginger and Bill Bercaw, Lisa and Ryan Cates, Jennifer and Brent Muhle, and Michele and Brian Smith, five lovely families whose homes were part of my research; to Doug Hosner, for all his help in putting this book into readable English; and to David Ensley, for reasons he knows.

ABOUT THE AUTHOR

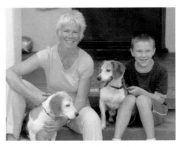

Penny Scott-Fox is one of the nation's most respected dog behavioral specialists. She works for the Pasadena Humane Society in Pasadena, California, and is a Fellow of the Pet Behavior Institute, Durham, England. Penny is an accomplished speaker, lecturing around the country for Emily Weiss Consulting on the SAFER behavior assessment for dogs in animal shelters. Aside from her very popular classes for dogs and their families, Penny's experience includes training shelter dogs and evaluating their behaviors. Using reward-based training, she has solved problem behaviors for hundreds of dogs. Her successful techniques have been covered by media outlets around the world, among them the Discovery Channel, CNN, Fox, French television, Japanese radio, the *Los Angeles Times,* and *People* magazine of Australia. In 2002, the United States Immigration and Naturalization Service bestowed on Ms. Scott-Fox the designation of "Alien of Extraordinary Ability." Only about 20 foreign nationals are so recognized each year.

ABOUT THE ILLUSTRATOR

For the past several decades, **Ingrid Kallick** has worked in print and electronic media and on murals and stage sets. Some of her credits include illustrations in the *Communication Arts Illustration Annual*, the cover of *Science*, and in *Scientific American.* Her current focus is on narrative illustration.